W9-BYK-378

NATURAL BEAUTY

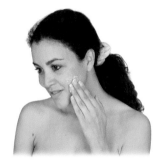

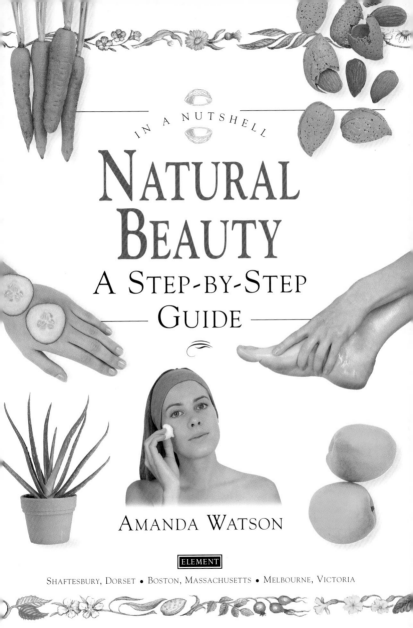

IN A NUTSHELL

NATURAL
BEAUTY
A STEP-BY-STEP
GUIDE

AMANDA WATSON

ELEMENT

SHAFTESBURY, DORSET • BOSTON, MASSACHUSETTS • MELBOURNE, VICTORIA

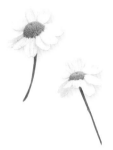

© Element Books Limited 1999

First published in Great Britain in 1999 by
ELEMENT BOOKS LIMITED
Shaftesbury, Dorset SP7 8BP

Published in the USA in 1999 by
ELEMENT BOOKS INC
160 North Washington Street,
Boston MA 02114

Published in Australia in 1999 by
ELEMENT BOOKS
and distributed by
Penguin Australia Ltd
487 Maroondah Highway,
Ringwood, Victoria 3134

All rights reserved.
No part of this book may be reproduced
or utilized in any form or by any means,
electronic or mechanical, without prior
permission in writing from the publisher.

NOTE FROM THE PUBLISHER
Any information given in this book is not
intended to be taken as a replacement for
medical advice. Any person with a
condition requiring medical attention
should consult a qualified practitioner or
therapist.

Designed and created for Element Books with
The Bridgewater Book Company Limited

ELEMENT BOOKS LIMITED
Creative Director Ed Day
Managing Editor Miranda Spicer
Senior Commissioning Editor Caro Ness
Editor Katie Worrall
Production Manager Susan Sutterby
Production Controller Claire Legg

THE BRIDGEWATER BOOK COMPANY
Art Director Sarah Howerd
Designer Jane Lanaway
Editorial Director Sophie Collins
Editor Nicky Adamson
Picture research Lynda Marshall
Three dimensional models Mark Jamieson
Photography Ian Parsons

Printed and bound in Singapore by
Tien Wah Press Pte Ltd.

Library of Congress Cataloging in Publication
DATA AVAILABLE

British Library Cataloging in Publication
data available

ISBN 1 86204 235 7

The publishers wish to thank the
following for the use of pictures:
Bridgeman Art Library, e.t.archive, Garden
Picture Library, Image Bank.

Special thanks go to:
Maria Andersson, C. Bayes, Maggie de Freitas,
Sara McGowan, Isobel Muston, Nick Muston,
Clare Pearson.

Special thanks go to:
Steamer Trading Cookshop, High Street,
Alfriston, East Sussex; Mackays Stores Ltd,
198 High Street, Lewes, East Sussex; Wyevale
Garden Centres plc, Newhaven Road,
Kingston nr. Lewes, East Sussex; Bright Ideas,
38 High Street, Lewes, East Sussex; for help
with properties.

Contents

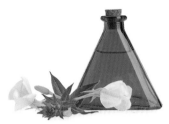

Discovering natural beauty

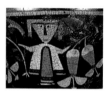

ABOVE **Healing plant lore transcends cultural borders.**

THE HEALING PROPERTIES of *flowers, plants, and fruits have been known since very early times. Natural beauty methods evolved through centuries of observation, trial, and error. Many cultures revered the healing properties of plants so deeply that they believed the plants to have magical powers as well.*

A sign of the importance attached to plants in ancient societies is that they were often buried alongside people in their tombs. Excavations in Iraq recently have revealed a 60,000-year-old burial site, in which eight different medicinal plants were found to have been buried.

The opening up of trade routes brought new plants and foodstuffs to different peoples. Knowledge of how to use new plants was spread by word of mouth over great distances, and recipes that have been handed down through the years are still with us today.

The soothing effect of oatmeal on the skin was discovered nearly 4,000 years ago.

ALMONDS

OATMEAL

APRICOTS

GERANIUM

RIGHT **Natural beauty products can benefit all skin types.**

Manufacturers of modern cosmetics are also aware of the advantage of using natural ingredients. Manufacturers, however, include chemical preservatives to lengthen the shelf-life of their products. In some cases, these chemicals mask the benefits of the natural ingredients, resulting in a cosmetic with only small quantities of active properties. Creating your own natural beauty preparations gives you the full benefit of undiluted amounts of nature's nutrients.

Discovering the vitamins, minerals, and enzymes found in natural ingredients and learning to put them to good use in beauty preparations will open up a world of possibilities for new ways to cleanse, nourish, and rejuvenate your skin and hair. In addition, producing an individual range, whether it be for yourself, or for your family and friends, is very rewarding.

ENZYMES

Enzymes are a protein substance found in living cells that bring about chemical changes. When used in beauty preparations, enzymes play an important role in breaking down surface bacteria, leaving the complexion glowing.

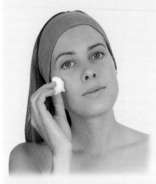

ABOVE **Skin toners can be based on natural products.**

RIGHT **Many everyday products can be used as beauty preparations.**

A brief history

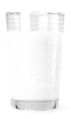

THE BENEFICIAL PROPERTIES *of natural substances have been harnessed in healing and health-giving preparations for use on the face and body since prehistoric times. Recently, scientists have established that many traditional beauty treatments really do work.*

ABOVE **Milk contains antiaging "fruit acids."**

Some of the earliest evidence of the widespread use of natural preparations to enhance beauty comes from ancient Egypt. Cleopatra (69–30 B.C.E.), the Egyptian queen, bathed in ass's milk to preserve her legendary beauty. Today we know that milk contains "fruit acids," currently being hailed as the most significant antiaging cosmetic discovery in years.

Two Greek physicians of the classical era – Hippocrates (c. 460–377 B.C.E.), known as the "father of medicine," and Galen (c. 130–201 C.E.) – left an important legacy. Hippocrates prescribed aromatic oils for health and Galen produced the first skin cream by mixing beeswax, olive oil, and rose water together.

ALOE VERA AND HONEY

Cleopatra used aloe vera as a skin cleanser. The Greeks and Romans called honey "ambrosia" and believed it was the food responsible for the immortality of the gods. Its rejuvenating properties can be harnessed in a number of natural beauty preparations.

LIQUID HONEY

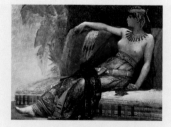

ABOVE **The benefits of honey as a beauty aid were well known in the ancient world.**

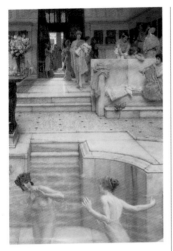

ABOVE *The Romans aspired to an ideal of natural beauty.*

The Romans, too, prided themselves on cleanliness and introduced bathhouses throughout Europe, which they scented with rose water and aromatic oils.

During the Middle Ages, "wise women" prescribed herbal remedies for skin care and beauty. The use of herbs during the centuries following the Middle Ages has been well documented. For example, Hungary water, the main ingredient of which is rosemary, was created in 1370. It was used by Queen Elizabeth of Hungary, who believed that washing in it removed wrinkles.

Aromatic oils, the oldest form of perfume known, were often heavily scented mixtures, used to mask unpleasant body odors. Although it was not considered fashionable to bathe in the days of Queen Elizabeth I of England (1533–1603), the queen herself knew the value of using herbal infusions to cleanse the skin.

Plants and other natural ingredients provided the fundamental materials for beauty preparations, perfumes, dyes, and medicines until the 20th century, when they were replaced by synthetics. But, despite the fact that modern cosmetology offers a wide range of synthetic products, many people are now choosing to use natural alternatives, drawing on wisdom that has been passed down from generation to generation.

RIGHT
Rosemary has been used since medieval times.

Beauty from within and without

ABOVE *Inner and outer beauty complement each other.*

OUTER BEAUTY *is the bloom of general health and well-being, in other words, inner beauty. To enhance your beauty, both inner and outer, you may simply need to set aside some stress-free time to relax and pamper yourself, or adapt your lifestyle in general. Whatever your particular situation, there are many natural ways to achieve beauty, from the inside out, and the outside in.*

DIET

A diet consisting of fried, refined, and preservative-laden food will take its toll on your appearance as well as your health. On the other hand, a good daily intake of fresh, organically grown vegetables and fruits will boost your immune system and improve your general health.

Water is one of nature's greatest natural cleansers, and drinking between six and eight glasses a day will improve the functioning of all your body's systems and help clear your complexion.

BELOW *Drinking plenty of water helps clear the system.*

LEFT *Good diet and regular exercise provide the basis for beauty.*

EXERCISE

Any form of exercise will help you feel and look better by relieving tension and stress. Exercising also helps the body get rid of excess stress hormones and toxins. Taking a healthy amount of exercise does not necessarily mean making disruptive changes to your routine, or buying expensive equipment. One of the most effective forms of exercise is walking, and the only equipment you need is a comfortable pair of shoes.

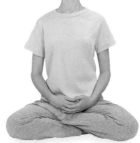

LEFT *Relaxation techniques such as yoga reduce stress.*

YOGA AND MEDITATION

Relaxation and peace of mind can be enhanced greatly by yoga and meditation. Both methods calm the mind and body to promote mental and physical well-being. Meditation, whether as a part of yoga, or used separately, aims to stop troubling or stimulating thoughts from entering the mind by focusing on the inhalation and exhalation of breath or by concentrating on a single neutral thought.

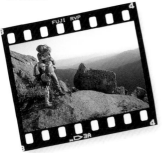

ABOVE *A country walk eases the mind and exercises the body.*

LEFT *Yoga combines meditation and body control.*

BATHING

Baths are an excellent time for pampering and relaxation, and you can create different atmospheres according to your needs. A few drops of a carefully chosen essential oil added to the water can be used to calm and relax, lift your spirits, or rejuvenate and energize. Using herbs in bathwater can also be highly beneficial – chamomile flowers, for example, act as a gentle nerve restorative.

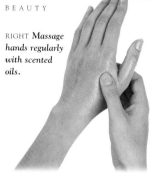

RIGHT *Massage hands regularly with scented oils.*

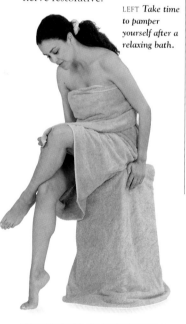

LEFT *Take time to pamper yourself after a relaxing bath.*

AROMATHERAPY MASSAGE

A potent combination of the healing powers of touch and essential oils, aromatherapy massage stimulates the circulation and promotes general health and well-being. Not only is it deeply relaxing, it can also eliminate toxins from the body, and help resolve such problems as back pain, tension, stiffness, and headaches.

The essential oils that form the basis of aromatherapy preparations also help to maintain the elasticity of the skin.

RIGHT *Tired feet benefit from the regular application of scented oils.*

SKIN BRUSHING

Brushing the skin stimulates the lymphatic system and the circulation. This action speeds the removal of toxic waste from the body, improving the overall condition of the skin. Using a natural bristle brush on dry skin (before you get into your shower or bath), begin by gently brushing the soles of the feet using firm, sweeping strokes always directed toward the heart. Continue brushing up the front of the legs and then the back, right up over the buttocks. Brush everywhere except your face and neck. Be gentle on the abdomen and breasts, avoiding the nipples. Follow with a shower or bath. A firmer brushing action may be used as long as you feel comfortable.

ABOVE *A skin brush should have natural bristles.*

LEFT *Brush the arms upward from the wrist.*

Brush is held flat

RIGHT *Brush legs from top of foot to knee, then from knee to hip.*

Use firm, sweeping strokes

CELLULITE

The dimpled "orange peel" skin that often occurs in women is known as cellulite. An accumulation of fluid and toxins in the fat cells, it can appear on the thighs, buttocks, upper arms, and stomach. Cellulite can be a result of hormonal imbalances, an unhealthy diet, lack of exercise, or stress. Massage, skin brushing, and the use of essential oils such as lemon, geranium, juniper, fennel, and rosemary all help. Every morning drink the juice of a lemon diluted in water, and drink fennel tea and plenty of water every day.

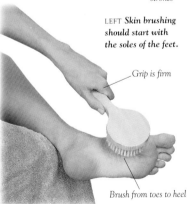

LEFT *Skin brushing should start with the soles of the feet.*

Grip is firm

Brush from toes to heel

Using essential oils

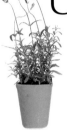

ESSENTIAL OILS *are extracted from aromatic plants and are best known as the basic tool of aromatherapy. Powerful and versatile, essential oils are highly effective in a broad range of beauty preparations. Many quite different essential oils blend well together and you can experiment with their aromas and complementary qualities. Essential oils are extremely concentrated, potent ingredients and must be used with care.*

ABOVE **Lavender** *essential oil is antiseptic and relaxing.*

Essential oils can be used in a number of different ways. Very few can be applied directly onto the skin and in most cases they must be diluted.

For external use, such as in a massage, blend 7 drops of essential oil in 1 tbsp (15 ml) of a carrier oil (*see page 16*).

Essential oils deteriorate rapidly after dilution so make sure that you mix only small quantities as you need them.

For a bath, add 6 drops of pure essential oil once the bathtub is full. Gently stir the water with your hand in order to disperse the droplets of oil.

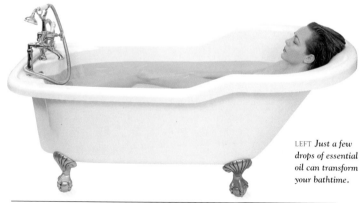

LEFT *Just a few drops of essential oil can transform your bathtime.*

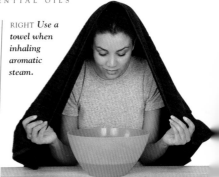

RIGHT *Use a towel when inhaling aromatic steam.*

CAUTIONS

If used in large quantities, essential oils can be toxic. Always read the instructions and, if in any doubt whatsoever, seek the advice of a qualified practitioner. Never use an essential oil internally unless instructed to do so by a professional practitioner. Herbs, too, should be used with care. Always consult a qualified aromatherapist or herbal practitioner in any of the following cases.

Consult a practitioner if:
• you are pregnant – some essential oils and certain herbs must be strictly avoided during pregnancy;
• you are receiving treatment for any medical condition, such as high blood pressure, epilepsy, or diabetes;
• you are treating babies and children.

If you have sensitive or particularly allergic skin always carry out a patch test (*see below*).

For a steam inhalation, 3 drops of essential oil added to 1 quart (1 liter) of freshly boiled water is sufficient. Cover your head and shoulders with a towel while you inhale to prevent the steam from dispersing.

For use in a face mask, 1–2 drops is enough.

BELOW *Cover a patch test area overnight to protect it.*

HOW TO DO A PATCH TEST

Apply a small amount of the substance you wish to test to the soft skin inside your wrist or elbow. Cover with a bandage and leave overnight. If any redness or irritation occurs, you may have a sensitivity to the substance and should avoid using it.

Using carrier oils

ESSENTIAL OILS are not used neat on the skin (with the exception of lavender and tea tree – unless you have very sensitive skin) but instead are diluted in a medium. When essential oils are to be used in a bath or facial sauna, they are diluted in water, but when they are to be used in massage, a carrier oil is used as a base. A carrier oil is a light vegetable- or plant-based oil. Sunflower, almond, apricot-kernel, avocado, grapeseed, jojoba, evening primrose, and wheat-germ oils all make excellent carrier oils. High-quality, cold-pressed oils will give maximum penetration of the skin.

ABOVE **Carrier oils are used to dilute powerful essential oils.**

Essential oils contain active constituents that are quickly absorbed, so using oils to treat oily skin will not make the skin more oily.

RIGHT **Carrier oils are pressed from a variety of nuts, kernels, and plants.**

CELLULITE TREATMENT

For a useful carrier oil for cellulite treatments, blend 2 tbsp (30 ml) of almond oil, 1 tsp (5 ml) of jojoba oil, and 5 drops of carrot oil.

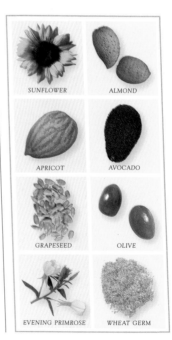

SUNFLOWER

ALMOND

APRICOT

AVOCADO

GRAPESEED

OLIVE

EVENING PRIMROSE

WHEAT GERM

CARRIER OILS USED ALONE

Some oils used as carrier oils in aromatherapy have their own beneficial properties, and can be used alone. Some important oils are listed, right.

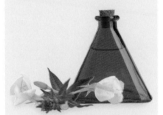

ABOVE *Oil derived from evening primrose has many beneficial properties.*

MASSAGE

Massage is one of the most powerful ways of introducing essential oils to the face and body.

Evening primrose oil is excellent for dry skin conditions and helps prevent premature aging. It is also helpful for dull or pale skin. It is best blended with another base oil.

Grapeseed oil is a light, easily absorbed oil most commonly used as a base oil; it can also be used on its own as a massage oil.

Jojoba oil is highly penetrative and suitable for all skin types. It can be used alone or mixed with another oil, and makes a good eye-makeup remover.

Olive oil has soothing and softening properties and is good for treating the scalp and dry hair (massage well into the scalp and hair). Soak very dry hands in olive oil for 30 minutes. The oil has quite a strong smell.

LEFT *Using oils during massage helps deep penetration into the skin.*

Masseur applies oils

Oil helps relaxation

Towel covers areas before and after massage

Natural beauty techniques

THERE ARE A NUMBER *of ways to apply homemade natural beauty preparations to your skin to maximize the benefits of the ingredients you have chosen. Different preparations suit different skin types. Specific recipes are listed later in the book.*

MAKING A FACE MASK

Face masks serve a wide range of purposes. Some masks can be used to cleanse and tone the skin, draw out impurities, clear blackheads, and soothe sore, inflamed acne. Others can be used to rejuvenate and restore the skin, or act as an intense, rehydrating moisturizer. They can also be used to exfoliate the skin, removing dead and damaged cells to reduce the development of wrinkles.

CAUTION

If you have sensitive skin, do a patch test before applying a face mask (see page 15).

Method: Recipes vary slightly. Mash 2 tsp of the main active ingredient (for example, banana or avocado). Blend with 1 tsp of a base (plain yogurt or honey). Spread over the face, avoiding the eye area and lips. Leave for 15 minutes and rinse off with water.

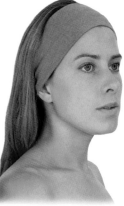

1 Whenever you apply a natural face mask be sure to tie your hair back and protect your clothing.

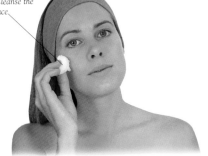

Cleanse the face

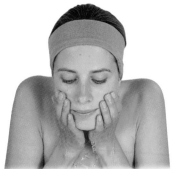

2 Cleanse the face thoroughly before applying a mask to remove bacteria and make-up.

4 Leave for 15 minutes and rinse off with water.

WATER

Surprisingly, water can dehydrate the skin. After rinsing off a face mask or body treatment, always moisturize the skin to ensure maximum nourishment and protection.

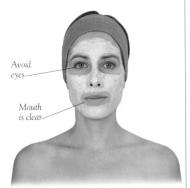

Avoid eyes

Mouth is clear

3 Prepare the mask thickly enough that the ingredients adhere to the skin, but not so thick that they pull on the skin when you apply them. Always avoid the lips and the area around the eyes when applying a face mask.

Skin is toned

Face feels restored

MAKING AN INFUSION

An infusion is an excellent way to use the more fragile aerial parts of leaves and flowers. Infusions are not just for drinking – they can be applied directly to the skin, blended with other ingredients, or inhaled with steam. Infusions can be used as cleansers, toners, or general skin-soothers. If you are using fresh flowers, bruise them slightly to release their oil.

Method: Use 1 cup (240 ml) of boiling water for each 1 tsp of dried herb or flower. If you are using fresh herbs or flowers, double the quantity to 2 tsp.

1 Fresh flowers should be slightly bruised before infusing, to help release their aromatic oils.

2 Pour the boiling water over the herbs or flowers and let stand for 10 minutes.

BELOW *Use dark-colored, light proof containers for storing preparations.*

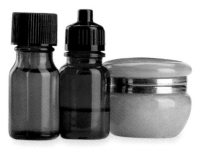

3 Strain and transfer to a glass bottle with a secure lid. Sealed, an infusion will keep up to 4 or 5 days in the refrigerator.

FACIAL SAUNA

A facial sauna is an effective way to cleanse the skin. The steam gently opens the pores and stimulates blood circulation, which clears the skin of toxins and helps prevent the buildup of acne. Additionally, the steam carries the chosen active ingredient from, for example, a flower, herb, or essential oil directly into the skin's pores.

> **CAUTION**
>
> Facial saunas are not recommended for those with sensitive skin or broken facial veins.

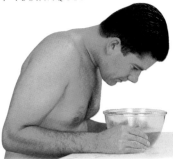

2 Sit over the bowl so you can feel your face absorbing the steam without discomfort.

1 Pour 1 quart (1 liter) of water that has just boiled into a large bowl. If using herbs or flowers (dried or fresh) pour the water on top of them. If using essential oils, add a few drops to the water.

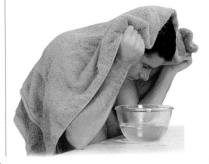

3 Cover your head and the bowl with a large towel to capture all the vapors. Relax for 10 minutes.

4 Splash your skin with cool water to close the pores, and pat dry.

Splash with cool water

Pat dry

Equipment and preparation

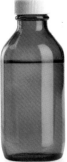

ABOVE *Ensure containers have tightly-fitting lids.*

YOU DO NOT NEED *to go out and buy any specialized, expensive, or complicated equipment in order to prepare your own treatments, but you do need to keep beauty utensils separate from food utensils. This will prevent bacteria or germs from cooking getting into your preparations.*

STERILIZATION AND HYGIENE

Bacteria will cause natural preparations to deteriorate quickly, so cleanliness is extremely important. Always begin by washing your hands. Sterilize any equipment with sterilizing tablets or fluids, following the instructions on the label. Keep all preparation surfaces clean and dry. To prevent the spread of germs, use a clean spoon or spatula instead of dipping your hands into the mixture.

USEFUL EQUIPMENT

- Opaque glass or plastic bottles and jars with tightly fitting lids
- Sharp knife, fork, spoon, whisk, spatula
- Metal measuring spoons
- Small bowls
- Plastic storage containers with lids
- Measuring cup
- Blender
- Sieve
- Cotton balls
- Sterilizing tablets or fluid
- Labels

LEFT *Many ordinary household utensils can be used for making beauty preparations.*

Storage

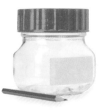

NATURAL BEAUTY REMEDIES *will last longer if they are stored in the refrigerator in tightly sealed containers, well away from any possible contamination by food. They should be clearly labelled.*

ABOVE *Label and date containers.*

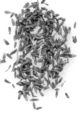

ABOVE *Keep herbs in airtight containers.*

STORING BEAUTY PREPARATIONS

Keeping any preparations in the refrigerator will help them last longer, but try to store them away from food to avoid spoilage. Essential oils and blends do not need to be refrigerated but should be kept in a cool place. Oils are sensitive to light and highly volatile so it is best to store them in dark bottles in a cupboard or drawer. Replace the lids immediately

after use. Fresh or dried herbs also need to be kept away from light. Store them in an airtight container to preserve their therapeutic properties.

Always label every item by name and date immediately after making it to avoid any confusion, especially if you are making more than one preparation at a time. You will also be able to keep track of the remedy's age.

BELOW *Store oils in a dark place such as a cupboard or drawer.*

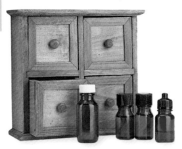

Save money by recycling storage containers. Any container that has a secure reusable lid, and can be sterilized, can be used again and again.

Preparation tips and guidelines

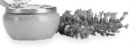

ABOVE **Prepare small quantities of fresh remedies.**

BY MAKING YOUR OWN *hair and skin care products, you can avoid the chemicals and preservatives found in commercial beauty products. However, fresh ingredients spoil very quickly and because your preparations do not contain any preservatives they will not last as long as commercial products. To get the best out of your beauty preparations, make only as much as you need each time.*

EXPERIMENT

Once you have been making your own preparations for a while, you can experiment. Either follow the recipes described, or look up the properties of a particular ingredient and prepare a recipe to suit your own skin type. Once you start creating different blends, you will see how easy it is to achieve results.

FRUITS AND VEGETABLES

When using fruits and vegetables, make sure they are as fresh as possible and thoroughly cleaned. Most store-bought produce today contains chemical pesticides, fungicides, and herbicides, so try to use organically grown produce instead, to get the best possible quality for your beauty remedies. Since homemade beauty preparations should be used up quickly to prevent deterioration, only small amounts of fresh ingredients are needed.

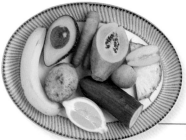

LEFT *Use organically grown fruit and vegetables to avoid contamination with chemicals.*

BASE CREAMS

You can buy pure base creams made from strictly natural ingredients to which you can add essential oils and other ingredients. Read the label to make sure that they do not contain perfume, color, or preservatives and that they are as pure as possible. This way, the base cream will not interfere with the therapeutic properties of the essential oils or any other ingredient you choose to blend into them. Pure base creams, not to be confused with preservative-laden synthetic cosmetics, can be purchased at a drugstore or health food outlet.

BELOW *Create flower waters from garden plants.*

FLOWER WATERS

Flower waters are distillations and infusions from essential oils and herbs, and they make refreshing skin tonics. Flower waters are often used in recipes instead of plain water, which may contain harmful additives.

COMMON FLOWER WATERS

Rose water is distilled from rose petals and makes an excellent, gentle toner for dry skin.
Orange flower water is a better choice for more oily skin because of its astringent properties.
Lavender water is a good toner for acne and is useful as a final rinse for oily hair.
Chamomile water is particularly calming and soothing for dry or sensitive skin.

The beauty aids

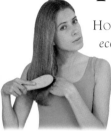

HOMEMADE PREPARATIONS *are natural, simple and economical to make. You decide on the ingredients you want to use – many of which can be found in the average kitchen. A remarkable number of everyday items, such as yogurt, eggs, and honey, can be put to good use on the skin and hair. Vegetables, fruits, herbs, flower waters, and oils all harbor a range of beneficial nutrients.*

ABOVE **Natural preparations enhance your normal grooming routine.**

This section gives a profile of the most useful ingredients in natural beauty preparations. In each case, the therapeutic properties of each beauty aid are given, along with suggestions for how to use the ingredients in preparations for face and body.

The condition of your skin changes from day to day. Making your own beauty preparations means you can easily adapt to daily needs without having to purchase new products. The measurements for "recipes" in this section have been kept as simple as possible. Some are given in American cups. An American cup is equivalent to 240 ml, just under half a British Imperial pint.

INGREDIENTS

All the ingredients mentioned in this book can be purchased from a grocery store, health food outlet, or herbal supplier. Always choose a reputable supplier – the highest-quality ingredients will produce the best results.

Tailor preparations to skin type

LEFT **Experiment with the rich variety of natural ingredients available.**

Banana

MUSA PARADISIACA SAPIENTUM

SLICED
BANANA

BENEFITS

Healing

Moisturizing

Nourishing

Soothing

THIS TROPICAL FRUIT *is full of vitamins and minerals that encourage a healthy skin tone. Bananas can be mashed easily to a paste for use on the skin and hair. With a high vitamin-C content, bananas promote the healing of acne and blemishes. Cut bananas turn brown very quickly but this does not hamper their effectiveness.*

RIGHT *Use fresh unbruised bananas for best results.*

BEAUTY RECIPES

To rehydrate dry skin, thoroughly mash enough banana to make 1 tbsp (20 g). Blend with 1 tsp of liquid honey and smooth all over a cleansed face and neck, avoiding the eye area. Relax for 20 minutes, then rinse off with warm water.

To untangle and nourish dry, frizzy, brittle hair, mash enough banana to make approximately ½ cup, depending on the length of your hair. Mix in enough grapeseed oil to make a smooth paste. Apply to the hair and cover with plastic wrap and a warm towel. Leave for one hour. Wash with a mild shampoo and rinse thoroughly. Can be used as often as once a week.

BELOW *Banana must be mashed to make a smooth paste.*

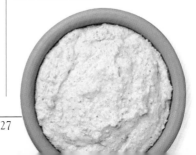

27

Avocado

PERSICA AMERICANA GRATISSMA

AVOCADO
STONE

Moisturizing
Nourishing
Rehydrating
Soothing

AVOCADOS ARE ONE *of the best natural cosmetic aids. Rich in vitamins A, B, C, and E, together with linoleic acid, lecithin, and natural plant oils, avocados contain many beneficial properties for promoting healthy skin and hair.*

BEAUTY RECIPES

For dry skin in need of rehydration and nourishment, mash enough ripe avocado to make 2 tsp, and blend with 1 tsp of plain, live yogurt and 1 tsp of liquid honey. Spread over the face, avoiding the eye area, and leave for 15 minutes before rinsing off with warm water.

To restore chemically damaged hair, mash half a small, ripe avocado and mix with 1 tsp (5 ml) of lemon juice. Apply thoroughly to the hair and cover with plastic wrap. Leave for one hour before washing out with a mild shampoo.

To remove rough skin, rub the insides of the avocado skin over the body. Rinse well and moisturize.

BELOW AND RIGHT
Ripe avocado flesh and liquid honey blend to make a rehydrating face mask.

Rub the avocado stone over your face before applying a face mask. This will stimulate pressure points and boost blood and lymphatic circulation, maximizing your skin's ability to absorb all the vitamins in the mask.

RIPE AVOCADO

LIQUID HONEY

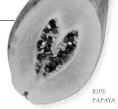

RIPE
PAPAYA

Papaya

CARICA PAPAYA

BENEFITS

Exfoliating
Healing
Rejuvenating

THIS TROPICAL FRUIT, *originally from Central America (and also known as papaw and pawpaw), contains an abundance of fruit enzymes. These enzymes help remove dead skin, a process known as exfoliation, aiding the healing of acne and blemishes. Enzyme exfoliation improves a dull complexion, making the skin look radiant and leaving a fresh, clean sensation.*

> **CAUTION**
>
> May irritate sensitive skin. Carry out a patch test (see page 15) before using.

BEAUTY RECIPES

✤ To remove dry, flaky skin, mash enough papaya to make 2 tsp, and mix in 1 tsp of liquid honey. Apply to the face and neck and leave for 15 minutes before rinsing. Follow with a moisturizer.

✤ To treat spots or acne, mash enough papaya to make 2 tsp and add 1 tsp of plain, live yogurt. Apply to the face and neck, avoiding the eyes and lips.

Leave for 15 minutes before rinsing with warm water.

✤ To reduce puffiness around the eyes, place very thin slices of papaya over closed eyelids. Leave for 5 minutes and rinse off with warm water.

✤ To remove dead skin cells and stimulate the circulation, rub the insides of the papaya skin all over the body. Rinse off.

LEFT *The papaya fruit has firm flesh and a core of seeds.*

LEFT *Mashed papaya can be used to make preparations for dry, flaky skin, and acne.*

Pineapple

ANANAS COMOSUS

PINEAPPLE SLICE

BENEFITS

Cleansing

Exfoliating

Rejuvenating

PINEAPPLE IS FULL of vitamins, minerals, and fruit enzymes and revitalizes the skin. It is also ideal for treating complexions troubled by oiliness or acne. An excellent cleanser, pineapple dissolves oil, dirt, and bacteria.

BEAUTY RECIPES

🌶 To revitalize the skin or to treat oiliness and acne, use the inside of a pineapple skin. Cut the skins to a size that can rest easily on the face and neck. Allow the pineapple to work for 10 to 15 minutes before rinsing with warm water. Finish with a moisturizer.

🌶 To soften hard cuticles on the hands or feet, blend a mixture of 2 tbsp (30 ml) of pineapple juice, 2 beaten egg yolks and 1 tsp (5 ml) of cider vinegar. Soak the nails in the mixture for 30 minutes. Rinse and dry thoroughly.

ABOVE **Peeled pineapple skin has revitalizing properties.**

Do not use on chapped hands: the solution may irritate the skin.

🌶 Constant contact with the enzymes in pineapple will gradually help dissolve a wart. Soak a small piece of absorbent cotton in fresh pineapple juice, or place a small piece of fresh pineapple against a wart and then wrap it in gauze or cheesecloth to keep it in place. Apply daily.

CAUTION

May irritate sensitive skin. Carry out a patch test (see page 15) before using.

RIGHT **Warts can be treated with fresh pineapple juice applied with absorbent cotton.**

30

Apple
MALUS SPECIES

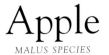

DESSERT APPLE

BENEFITS

Cooling

Exfoliating

Healing

Rejuvenating

Toning

APPLE CONTAINS *enzymes that help shed dead skin cells and bacteria to clear a complexion troubled with boils and acne. It helps restore the skin's acidity, protecting it from infection. As well as being rich in essential minerals, apples also contain vitamins A and C, which help the growth and repair of body tissue cells.*

BEAUTY RECIPES

❋ To make a toning mask for combination skin, blend 2 apples to a juice, smooth over the face, and leave for 15 to 20 minutes. Rinse thoroughly and moisturize.

❋ To treat acne, slice an apple thinly and gently stew it in a little water. When the apple is soft, let it stand until cool enough to smooth over the face. Leave it for 15 minutes, then rinse off.

❋ In cases of dandruff, combine 2 tbsp (30 ml) each of pure apple juice and warm water and massage into the scalp. Leave for 10 minutes, then wash the hair. Repeat 2 or 3 times a week.

❋ To treat sunburn, apply slices of apple to cool the skin and help reduce inflammation.

Throughout history the apple has been considered a sacred fruit of health and prosperity.

ABOVE **Slices of apple help sunburn.**

Smooth stewed apple over face

Protects skin from infection and kills bacteria

LEFT **Stewed apple provides a gentle balm for acne.**

ABOVE **Apple is effective in the treatment of skin infections.**

Cucumber

CUCUMIS SATIVUS

SLICED
CUCUMBER

Cleansing
Soothing
Toning

THE SKIN OF THE CUCUMBER *contains most of the vitamins and minerals, so it is best used unpeeled. Rich in vitamin C, cucumber applied to the skin will break down bacteria, making the complexion less susceptible to acne. Cucumber also contains potassium, silicon, and sulfur, which keep skin cells healthy and help maintain elasticity.*

BEAUTY RECIPES

🌿 To help soothe tired, irritated, puffy eyes and reduce swelling, lie down and place thin slices of cucumber over the eyelids. An ideal time might be while you are using a face mask. Relax for 15 minutes, then rinse off with cool water.

🌿 To make a toner to close enlarged pores, pulp half a medium-size cucumber (250 g) in a blender. Add 1 tbsp (15 ml) of witch hazel and 1 tsp (5 ml) of mineral or lavender water. Strain through a sieve. Pat onto the face and leave for 5 minutes. Rinse off with warm water before moisturizing. This toner will keep for 2 to 3 days if refrigerated.

🌿 For an effective astringent for acne, blend half a medium-size cucumber (250 g) and mix with 1 tsp (5 ml) of lemon juice. Smear over the face and leave for 5 minutes before rinsing.

Thin cucumber slices

Slice is laid flat

LEFT
Cucumber slices can be used to soothe mild sunburn.

WHOLE CUCUMBER

Potato

SOLANUM TUBEROSUM

ORGANIC
POTATOES

BENEFITS
Anti-
inflammatory
Softening
Soothing

THE POTATO IS *a major source of B vitamins, which help reduce facial oiliness and blackhead formation. To use it, slice raw potato very thinly, or grate or juice it. There is no need to peel the potato.*

BEAUTY RECIPES

❧ For an inflamed, pimply complexion, extract the juice from 4 small potatoes (pulp them in a blender) and combine with 1–2 tsp (5–10 g) of finely ground oatmeal to form a paste. Gently rub into the skin for a few minutes, then leave for 15 minutes before rinsing with warm water.

❧ To relieve puffy, swollen eyes, place a very thin slice of potato on each closed eye. Relax for 15 minutes, then remove the potato and wash off its juice with cool water. You can combine this treatment with a face mask.

❧ To treat sunburn, apply thin slices of potato or a thin layer of grated potato to cool the skin and help reduce inflammation.

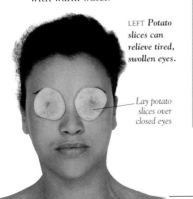

LEFT **Potato slices can relieve tired, swollen eyes.**

Lay potato slices over closed eyes

RIGHT
Grated potato will relieve sunburn.

Carrot

DAUCUS CAROTA

Antiaging
Cleansing
Moisturizing
Nourishing

CARROTS ARE RICH *in vitamins A, B, C, and beta-carotene. These help keep the skin, hair, and eyes healthy. Carrots suit an oily, pimply skin as well as dry skin. Carrot oil, which can be purchased in health food stores, helps reduce scarring.*

BEAUTY RECIPES

❈ To heal pimples and boils, or to ease sunburn, grate a medium-sized carrot (120 g). For pimples and boils, but not for sunburn, mix in 1 tsp (5 ml) of lemon juice. Pat gently onto the face and relax for 5 minutes, but no longer because the carrot may stain the skin if left on too long. Rinse off with warm water and moisturize.

❈ To soothe inflamed skin, finely grate a medium-sized carrot (120 g), add 1 tbsp plain, live yogurt and mix thoroughly. Chill in the refrigerator for several hours. Smooth onto the skin and leave for 10 minutes. Rinse and pat dry.

RAW CARROTS

❈ To rejuvenate and moisturize the skin, blend 5 drops of pure carrot oil with 1 tsp (5 ml) of a carrier oil and massage well into the skin. If acne is present, blend in a few drops of wheat-germ oil as well before applying to skin.

RIGHT *Use carrot oil to reduce scarring.*

CAUTION

Do not use carrot oil undiluted on the skin, because it may briefly stain it. Always blend with another carrier oil.

Almond

PRUNUS AMYGDALUS

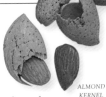

ALMOND
KERNEL

BENEFITS
Exfoliating
Nourishing
Softening

THE EMOLLIENT PROPERTIES of *almonds make them very suitable for cosmetic use. Ground almonds are good as a gently abrasive body and facial scrub, and the oil is very soothing.*

BEAUTY RECIPES

❧ To make a scrub to remove flaky skin, mix 1 tbsp (10 g) of ground almonds with 1 tbsp of oatmeal and add enough flower water (*see page 25*) to make a paste. Gently rub into the face, concentrating on problem areas. Make up larger quantities for a body scrub.

❧ For dry and damaged hair, combine 2 tbsp (30 ml) of almond oil and 1 tsp of liquid honey and beat in 1 egg yolk. Massage well into the scalp, then cover the hair with plastic wrap and a warm towel. For best results leave overnight and rinse out with a mild shampoo.

❧ For dry skin, massage a few drops of almond oil into the face and neck after cleansing at night. This method is also good for dry, chapped hands.

❧ To revitalize dull, pale skin, combine 1 tbsp (10 g) of ground almonds with enough almond oil to make a smooth paste and apply thoroughly to the face and neck. Gently rub over the skin for a few minutes, then leave the almond paste in place for 15 minutes. Rinse thoroughly.

CAUTION

Almonds should be avoided by those allergic to nuts.

LEFT *Blend ground almonds with almond oil for a face mask.*

Apricot

PRUNUS ARMENIACA

BENEFITS
Moisturizing
Nourishing
Revitalizing

APRICOTS CAN BE USED *to make a refreshing facial remedy, and can be combined with other fruits or ingredients for an invigorating treatment. Apricot oil is extracted from the kernel of the fruit and contains vitamins and minerals that make it particularly suitable for dry, sensitive skin.*

APRICOTS

BEAUTY RECIPES

🌸 For a softening mask for dry skin, peel 2 fresh apricots and mash the fruit to a smooth pulp. Mix with 1 tsp (5 ml) of avocado oil to make a paste. Spread onto the face and leave for 15 minutes. Rinse and moisturize.

🌸 For wrinkles, combine 1 tbsp (15 ml) each of the oils of apricot kernel, almond, and wheat germ in a screwtop jar and shake thoroughly. Dab a little oil on the delicate skin around the eyes. This is best done daily, last thing at night after cleansing.

🌸 Make your own eye-makeup remover pads by using 1 tbsp (15 ml) of apricot-kernel oil, and 1 tbsp (15 ml) of rose water. Soak cotton balls in the mixture and keep in a sealed container ready for use.

RIGHT **Apricots make useful preparations for the face.**

RIGHT **The apricot kernel provides the carrier oil.**

LEMON
SEGMENT

Lemon

CITRUS LIMON

BENEFITS

Antiseptic

Astringent

Mild bleaching
properties

Rejuvenating

Stimulating

CONTAINING CITRIC ACID, *lemon restores
the natural acid balance of the skin. Lemons
are rich in vitamin C, which helps maintain the
collagen needed for healthy skin and hair. Vitamin
C also helps to counteract infection
and is therefore ideal for greasy skin.*

CAUTION

Citrus oils may
irritate sensitive
skins. Use only a few
drops at a time.
Do not use before
going out in the sun
or sunbeds.
Do not use lemon
juice on sore or
irritated skin.

BEAUTY RECIPES

❊ For oily skin, make a simple
toner by diluting 1 tbsp (15 ml)
of lemon juice in 2 cups (500 ml)
of distilled water.
Wipe over the
face using a
cotton ball after
cleansing. Make
a fresh batch
each day in order to
prevent bacterial growth.

LEFT *Lemons
have both
antiseptic
and
astringent
properties.*

❊ For oily hair, squeeze
the juice of 2 lemons into
1 quart (1 liter) of distilled
water and rinse the hair
repeatedly with the liquid
until it has all been used.

❊ To treat dandruff, rub the
juice of 1 lemon thoroughly into
the scalp. Leave for 10 minutes
before rinsing.

❊ To remove discolored or hard
skin on elbows, rub the elbows
with lemon halves.

ESSENTIAL OIL

❧ For cellulite add 5 drops to
2 tbsp (30 ml) of carrier oil
(*see page 16*) and massage the
whole body.

❧ For a refreshing, invigorating
bath, use 2 or 3 drops in the bathwater.

Sandalwood

SANTALUM ALBUM

BENEFITS

Antiseptic

Astringent

Regenerative

Rehydrating

Soothing

THIS ESSENTIAL OIL *is extracted from the heartwood of the sandalwood tree and has a sweet, heady, wood-scented aroma. It is beneficial for both oily and dry skin types. Widely reputed to be an aphrodisiac, its sensual aroma is popular with both men and women.*

BEAUTY RECIPES

❧ For a dry or oily complexion, add 3 drops of sandalwood to 2 tsp (10 ml) of jojoba oil and massage thoroughly into the face at night after cleansing.

❧ For oily skin, make a facial sauna (*see page 21*) by adding 2 or 3 drops to a bowl of hot water.

❧ For dry, cracked hands or feet, add 7 drops of sandalwood to 1 tbsp (15 ml) of almond oil and massage thoroughly into the skin. Use nightly before going to sleep.

❧ For chapped skin, add 7 drops of sandalwood oil to the bath.

Sandalwood has been used for many centuries in India and is still widely used today in perfumes, soaps, and cosmetics.

LEFT *Sandalwood oil is extracted from the heartwood and roots.*

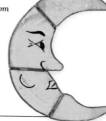

RIGHT *Bedtime is the most convenient time to apply greasy oils.*

Geranium

PELARGONIUM GRAVEOLENS

BENEFITS
Antiseptic
Astringent
Balancing
Diuretic
Stimulating

GERANIUM ESSENTIAL OIL *has a delightful, uplifting fragrance. Its ability to balance the secretion of sebum makes it valuable for combination complexions or skin that is very dry or very oily. It has a stimulating effect on the lymphatic system and can be added to carrier oils for treating cellulite.*

GERANIUM FLOWER AND LEAF

BEAUTY RECIPES

❉ For combination skin, blend 3 drops of geranium with 2 tsp (10 ml) of jojoba oil and use as an effective moisturizer after cleansing the skin at night.

Lymph nodes

Lymph vessels

LEFT *The lymphatic system carries waste from the body's cells.*

❉ For dry or oily skin, make a facial sauna (*see page 21*) by adding 2 or 3 drops of geranium essential oil to a bowl of hot water.

❉ For cellulite, use 6 drops in the bath or make an all-over body massage blend by adding 15 drops to 2 tbsp (30 ml) of carrier oil (*see page 16*).

Sebum is the oil secreted by the sebaceous glands. It acts as a lubricant for the skin and hair and provides some protection against bacteria.

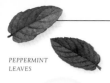
PEPPERMINT
LEAVES

Peppermint

MENTHA PIPERITA

BENEFITS

Analgesic
Anti-inflammatory
Cooling
Invigorating

PEPPERMINT IS A *stimulating plant with mild antiseptic and antibacterial properties that help control bacteria on the skin's surface. It is also good for easing aches and pains. The herb and the essential oil are both used in beauty preparations.*

BEAUTY RECIPES

❀ To cleanse the skin, encourage the circulation of blood, and help prevent the buildup of acne, steam the face with peppermint. Make an infusion of the peppermint herb and add to a facial sauna (*see page 21*). Steam the face for 5 to 10 minutes and then splash the face with cold water. Finish with a moisturizer.

BELOW *A mint infusion soothes tired feet.*

CAUTION

Use only a few drops of essential oil at a time. Do not use during the first three months of pregnancy or when taking homeopathic remedies. Do not use in the evening, since it may cause wakefulness.

RIGHT
Peppermint is easy to grow in a garden or window box.

ESSENTIAL OIL

❦ To refresh tired, aching legs, add 2 drops to 1 tbsp (15 ml) of grape-seed oil and massage into the legs starting from the ankles and working toward the buttocks.

❦ To soothe hot, throbbing feet, add 1 drop to a bowl of warm water and soak the feet for 10 minutes. Dry the feet and wrap them in a warm towel for 5 minutes, then massage using wheat-germ oil.

Tea tree

MELALEUCA ALTERNIFOLIA

BENEFITS

Antibacterial
Antifungal
Antiseptic

THE ABORIGINAL PEOPLE *of Australia have been using the healing force of tea tree for centuries and it is now one of Australia's significant exports. Used in combating infectious organisms, the essential oil is ideal for many skin problems.*

BEAUTY RECIPES

❀ To treat pimples, boils, and cold sores, place 1 drop of tea tree essential oil onto a Q-tip and apply directly to the aggravated area. Or add 1 drop to any face mask or scrub. Alternatively, you can make a facial sauna (*see page 21*) by adding 2 drops to a bowl of hot water.

BELOW *Tea tree oil is distilled from the leaves and twigs.*

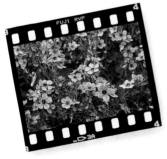

❀ To treat dandruff, blend 4 tbsp (60 ml) of jojoba oil with 30 drops of tea tree oil and massage into the scalp 3 times a week.

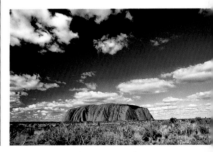

ABOVE *Ayres Rock in Australia. Tea tree is native to the Australian continent.*

This is one of the very few oils that can be used neat. However, if you have particularly sensitive skin, do a patch test first (*see page 15*).

Juniper

JUNIPERUS COMMUNIS

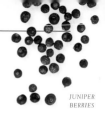

JUNIPER
BERRIES

BENEFITS

Antiseptic
Astringent
Diuretic
Purifying
Tonic

THE CLEANSING PROPERTIES *of the essential oil of juniper are beneficial for oily skin and are particularly detoxifying for the body. Combined with other detoxifying oils, a cleansing diet, skin brushing, and exercise, juniper can play an important role in dealing with cellulite.*

BEAUTY RECIPES

🌾 To cleanse greasy skin or skin that is prone to acne, use juniper in a facial sauna (*see page 21*) by adding 3 drops to a bowl of hot water.

LEFT *Juniper essential oil is extracted from berries, needles, and wood.*

🌾 To ease water retention before a period, add 6 drops to a warm bath.

🌾 For treating cellulite, add 3 drops of juniper and 3 drops of fennel essential oils to a bath and relax for at least 10 minutes. You can also add 15 drops of juniper essential oil to 2 tbsp (30 ml) of carrier oil (*see page 16*) and massage the entire body. Alternatively, add 10 drops of juniper to 2 tbsp (30 ml) of base cream or lotion to use on the body.

RIGHT
Stretching exercises help to disperse cellulite in thighs.

Knee is straight

Foot pulled back

CAUTION

Do not use juniper essential oil during pregnancy.

Fennel

FOENICULUM VULGARE

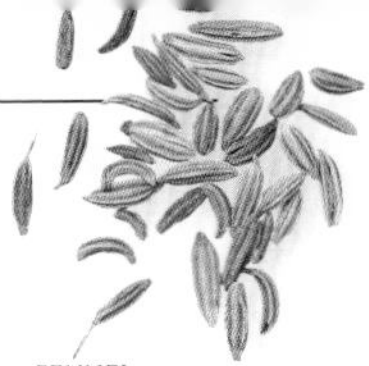

FENNEL SEEDS

BENEFITS

Antiseptic
Cleansing
Detoxifying
Restorative

FENNEL HAS BEEN *used since very early days for its curative effects. It contains an estrogen-like substance that helps maintain the elasticity of the skin. The herb, the seed, and the essential oil can all be used in beauty preparations.*

CAUTION

Fennel essential oil should not be used by people with epilepsy, children under six years of age, or during pregnancy.

BEAUTY RECIPES

For a soothing, antiwrinkle mask, make a strong infusion (*see page* 20) of the herb or seed. Add 2 tsp (10 ml) to 1 tsp of liquid honey and 1 tsp plain, live yogurt to make a smooth paste. Spread over the face and neck and leave for 20 minutes before rinsing.

To relieve tired, puffy eyes, soak 2 cotton balls in a fennel infusion and apply to closed eyes while relaxing with a face mask.

To treat cellulite, make a pot of tea by steeping 2 tsp of fennel seeds in ½ quart (½ liter) of boiling water. Drink one pot daily.

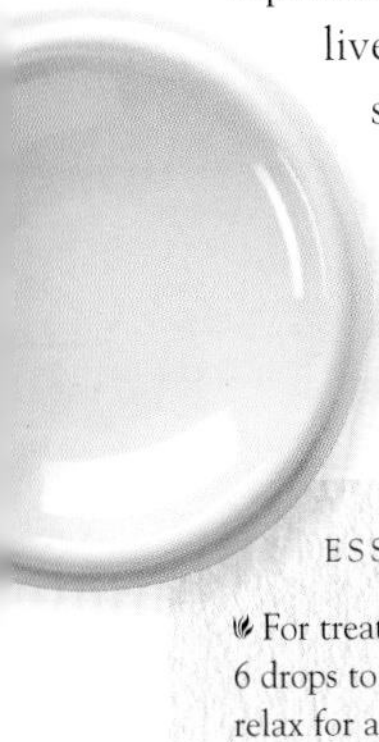

LEFT ***Fennel essential oil may help eliminate cellulite.***

ESSENTIAL OIL

For treating cellulite, add 6 drops to a warm bath and relax for at least 10 minutes. Alternatively, add 15 drops to 2 tbsp (30 ml) of the cellulite base oil (*see page* 16) and massage the whole body.

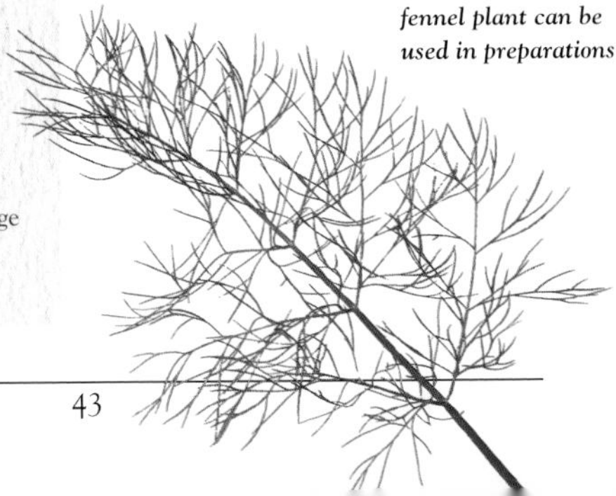

LEFT ***All parts of the fennel plant can be used in preparations.***

Rosemary

ROSMARINUS OFFICINALIS

ROSEMARY

BENEFITS
Antiseptic
Astringent
Detoxifying
Stimulating

ROSEMARY IS PROBABLY one of the most popular and widely used aromatic plants. It improves the circulation and is effective as a treatment for hair loss or hair that is in poor condition. Rosemary cleanses the skin deeply by opening the pores and ridding the skin of impurities. Both the herb and the essential oil are useful, particularly for oily skin.

BEAUTY RECIPES

❊ To relax and revive puffy, swollen eyes, lie down for 15 minutes with a cold rosemary tea bag on each closed eye.

❊ To restore color or add shine to dark hair, use an infusion of rosemary as a final rinse.

❊ To strengthen the hair and eliminate dandruff or improve dull, lank hair, massage an infusion of dried rosemary into the scalp after shampooing.

❊ For an oily complexion, use a rosemary infusion (*see page 20*) to tone.

LEFT **Rosemary needles dry easily so you could use your own plants.**

BELOW **Cold, infused rosemary tea bags help tired eyes.**

CAUTION

Do not use rosemary essential oil during pregnancy. It is not suitable for people with epilepsy or high blood pressure.

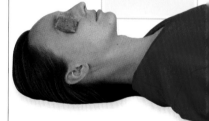

ESSENTIAL OIL

❧ For greasy skin or skin that is prone to acne, make a facial sauna (*see page 21*) by adding 2 drops to a bowl of hot water.

❧ For cellulite, use rosemary in a massage. Blend 2 tbsp (30 ml) of almond oil with 15 drops and massage over the body. Or, add 6 drops to bathwater.

Chamomile

CHAMOMILLA RECUTITA

CHAMOMILE
FLOWERS

BENEFITS
Anti-
inflammatory
Calming
Soothing

THERE ARE MANY *varieties of this well-known plant. Chamomile is valuable for skin problems, particularly where the skin is dry, flaky, or itchy. Famous for its mild bleaching properties that add golden highlights to fair hair, the herb and the essential oil are both used in beauty preparations.*

BEAUTY RECIPES

❋ To unclog the pores and treat blackheads, steam the face with an infusion of chamomile flowers (*see page 20*) for 10 minutes. Follow with a facial scrub and then moisturize.

❋ To relax and revive puffy, swollen, or tired eyes, lie down for 15 minutes with cold chamomile tea bags placed on each closed eye.

CAUTION

Do not use chamomile essential oil during the first three months of pregnancy, or at all during pregnancy if there is any history of miscarriages or complications.

❋ To add shine to fair hair, make an infusion of chamomile flowers with 1 quart (1 liter) of water (*see page 20*). Rinse hair thoroughly after shampooing.

❋ For a relaxing bath, infuse 4 or 5 handfuls of dried chamomile flowers for 10 minutes. Strain; add to bath.

ABOVE *Chamomile flowers infusing in hot water to create a hair rinse.*

ESSENTIAL OIL

❦ To relieve dry, sensitive skin on the face, add 3 drops to 2 tsp (10 ml) of apricot-kernel oil and massage into the skin after cleansing.

❦ To calm flaky, itchy skin, add 6 drops to a warm bath and soak for at least 10 minutes.

RIGHT *Chamomile may be used to treat blocked pores.*

Lavender

LAVANDULA VERA

LAVENDER OIL

BENEFITS

Anti-inflammatory

Antiseptic

Balancing

Relaxing

Soothing

A WELL-KNOWN FLOWER, *famous for its aroma and healing properties, lavender is valuable in natural beauty remedies. It has the ability to normalize the secretions of the sebaceous glands, benefiting both dry or oily skin. Lavender inhibits bacteria and stimulates the growth of healthy new cells.*

BEAUTY RECIPES

For a refreshing skin tonic for dry or oily skin, combine a handful of lavender flowers with 1 cup (240 ml) of apple cider vinegar in a screwtop jar. Add 3 cups (720 ml) of rose water and let the flowers steep for a week. Shake once a day. Strain and use daily on a cotton ball. Store in the refrigerator.

For rough hands, combine 1 tbsp (15 ml) of almond oil with 7 drops of lavender oil and massage in.

RIGHT **Lavender essential oil is produced from the flowers.**

CAUTION

Do not use during the first three months of pregnancy, or at all during pregnancy if there is any history of miscarriages or complications.

BELOW **Massage rough or chapped hands with lavender and almond oil.**

ESSENTIAL OILS

This is one of the very few oils that can be used neat. Apply 1 drop directly onto a pimple, spot, or boil to heal the infection.

To treat acne, you can make a facial sauna (*see page 21*) by adding 2 drops to a bowl of hot water.

To relieve tension in the feet and soften hard skin at the same time, add a few drops of lavender oil to a footbath and soak the feet for 10 minutes.

Wheat germ

THIS FOOD SUPPLEMENT *is one of the richest known sources of vitamin E. The oil has a strong, nutty aroma, is very nourishing for dry, sensitive skin, and helps reduce scarring. It is also a natural antioxidant, which means that when blended with other oils it helps stop them from becoming rancid; it also makes them last.*

BENEFITS
Exfoliating
Healing
Moisturizing

BEAUTY RECIPES

* For dry, patchy skin, mix together 1 tsp (2.5 g) of wheat germ, 2 tsp (10 ml) of liquid honey, 1 tsp (5 ml) of lemon juice, and 1 tsp (5 ml) of almond oil to form a paste. Gently massage into the face and neck for a few minutes, avoiding the eye area. Leave for 10 minutes, before rinsing well and moisturizing.

Wheat-germ oil is highly concentrated. If you find it is too thick, blend it with other carrier oils (see page 16).

RIGHT **Wheat-germ oil may prevent acne scarring.**

* To help reduce possible scarring caused by severe acne, massage a few drops of wheat-germ oil into the skin after cleansing at night. Use daily.

* To treat dry or heat-damaged hair, use enough wheat-germ oil to cover the whole of the scalp and massage in thoroughly. Cover the hair with plastic wrap and then a warm towel, and leave on overnight. Wash the hair with a mild shampoo. To remove oils from the hair, thoroughly massage a gentle shampoo into the hair and scalp before using water. When the oil has dispersed, rinse with water and if necessary repeat.

ABOVE **Wheat germ can be used in face and body scrubs.**

Honey

BENEFITS
Antibacterial
Cleansing
Moisturizing
Nourishing
Soothing

SINCE ANCIENT TIMES *honey has been used for its rejuvenating powers. Rich in minerals and vitamins, it attracts and retains fluids and acts as a moisturizer on the skin. Honey contains an antibacterial agent called inhibane, which promotes healing. Liquid honey is easier to use in beauty recipes than other, thicker honeys, and will help bind other materials to the skin.*

ABOVE *Use liquid honey for preparations.*

BEAUTY RECIPES

❋ To cleanse the skin, combine 1 tbsp (15 ml) of liquid honey and 1 tsp (5 ml) of wheat-germ oil with 3 drops of apricot-kernel oil. Add 1 tsp (5 ml) of flower water and mix well. Smooth over the face and neck and leave for 10 minutes. Wet a facecloth in warm water and wring it out. Gently remove the facial mixture by wiping with the warm facecloth.

❋ To heal sore or dry lips, melt 1 tbsp (15 ml) of liquid honey and stir in 1 tsp (5 ml) of rose water. Transfer to a small jar and seal. Use as a lip balm.

❋ To soften dry skin on elbows and knees, warm 2 tbsp (30 ml) of honey and rub into the skin. Leave for 20 minutes. Rinse off and pat dry.

BELOW *Honey has long been valued for its healing powers.*

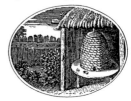

LEFT *Apply warmed honey to soften dry skin on elbows.*

Apple cider vinegar

ACETIC ACID

BENEFITS

Antiseptic

Astringent

Soothing

THERE ARE MANY *types of vinegars available, but apple cider vinegar is more suited to skin care. It helps restore the acidity of the skin, which protects it from infection. Cider vinegar softens the skin and is a useful beauty aid for the hair and scalp.*

ABOVE **Vinegar made from apples is ideal for beauty treatments.**

BEAUTY RECIPES

❧ To freshen and hydrate the skin and to remove any remaining dirt, soap, or cleanser, add 1 tsp (5 ml) of cider vinegar to 1 cup (240 ml) of water. Mix thoroughly and use as a toner after cleansing the skin. Keep refrigerated in a sealed jar and use within a week.

❧ The natural pH balance of the hair can be upset by piped water and shampoos. Use cider vinegar to help restore the pH balance and the condition of hair. Add 2 tbsp (30 ml) of cider vinegar to 1 quart (1 liter) of warm water and use to rinse hair after shampooing.

❧ To relieve dry, itchy skin, add 1 cup (240 ml) of cider vinegar to your bathwater.

❧ To strengthen weak, brittle nails, soak them for 5 to 10 minutes in enough cider vinegar to cover the nails. Avoid broken skin.

Hair has been washed

LEFT **A cider vinegar rinse helps restore pH balance in the hair.**

Apply rinse directly

CAUTION

Vinegar could irritate sensitive skin, so do a patch test first (see *page 15*).

49

Eggs

BENEFITS

Astringent
Conditioning
Nourishing

FULL OF *vitamins, protein, iron, and lecithin, eggs are inexpensive and versatile. Egg whites are useful for oily or blemished skin. Yolks make enriching face masks and shampoos. The whole egg can be used for hair conditioners. Do not use hot ingredients with eggs, or they will cook.*

EGGS

BEAUTY RECIPES

For a mask to treat dry skin, stir an egg yolk into 5 drops of wheat-germ oil and 1 tsp (5 ml) of warm honey. Apply to the face and leave for 10 to 15 minutes before rinsing and moisturizing.

LEFT **Dry skin may be treated with egg yolk, wheat-germ oil, and honey.**

LEMON

RIGHT **Treat oily skin with egg white, lemon, and witch hazel.**

WITCH HAZEL

To treat oily skin, mix an egg white with 5 drops of witch hazel and 1 tsp (5 ml) of lemon juice. Smooth over the face and neck. Leave for 10 minutes, then rinse well and moisturize.

For a quick remoisturizing treatment for dry hair, whisk 2 eggs into $\frac{1}{2}$ cup (120 ml) of warm water and massage well into the hair and scalp. Leave for 10 minutes before rinsing.

To condition dry hair, warm 2 tsp of honey. In a separate bowl, beat 1 egg yolk with 1 tbsp (15 ml) of cider vinegar. Remove the honey from the heat and slowly combine the two mixtures. Apply to the hair and cover with plastic wrap and then a warm towel. Leave for an hour, then shampoo and rinse.

Yogurt

BENEFITS
Cleansing
Moisturizing
Nourishing

A HIGHLY EFFECTIVE *beauty aid*, *yogurt can be used in face and body masks and hair conditioners. Always choose plain, live yogurt. "Live" means it contains bacteria-destroying enzymes which can help skin that is prone to acne.*

PLAIN YOGURT

BEAUTY RECIPES

For a soothing and healing mask for oily skin and skin prone to acne, mix 2 tbsp (40 g) of yogurt with 1 beaten egg white and enough finely ground oatmeal to form a thick paste. Apply to the face and neck and leave for 10 to 15 minutes. Rinse with warm water.

For a good conditioner for oily or uncontrollable hair, whisk ½ cup (160 g) of yogurt with 1 egg and massage into the hair after shampooing. Leave for 10 minutes and rinse thoroughly.

ABOVE *Use a hand whisk to blend yogurt.*

To relieve sunburn, combine ½ cup (160 g) of yogurt with 2 tbsp (30 ml) of rose water. Apply to the affected areas. Leave for 10 minutes then rinse. Use immediately, because it will not keep.

To soften hard, discolored skin on the feet, mix together ½ cup (160 ml) of yogurt with 1 tsp (5 ml) of cider vinegar. Smooth all over the feet and leave for 10 minutes before rinsing well.

ABOVE *Rose water with yogurt can relieve sunburn.*

LEFT *A yogurt and oatmeal face pack helps oily skin.*

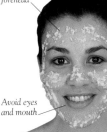

Face pack applied to forehead

Avoid eyes and mouth

Oatmeal

AVENA PATIVA

BENEFITS
Exceptionally
healing
Exfoliating
Soothing

OATS HAVE LONG *been known for their skin-soothing properties. Oatmeal is ground from whole oats and can be bought in fine, medium, and coarse meal. Finely-ground oatmeal acts as a gentle abrasive and is ideal for face and neck masks. Medium and coarse oatmeal make excellent exfoliating body scrubs.*

A RIPE EAR OF OATS

BEAUTY RECIPES

❋ To exfoliate rough, flaky facial skin, combine 2 tsp of fine oatmeal and 2 tsp of ground almonds. Add 1–2 tsp (5–10 ml) of cider vinegar and 1 drop of sandalwood oil and mix well. Gently rub into the skin for a few moments and rinse. For an all-over body scrub, increase the quantities and use medium or coarse oatmeal. Moisturize with oil or cream.

❋ To soothe dry skin, add a cupful of oatmeal (100 g) to a warm bath and soak for 10 minutes. Shower or rinse afterward to remove the oatmeal from the skin.

DEEP TREATMENT

After exfoliating and moisturizing the hands and feet, cover them with plastic wrap, slip on some cotton gloves or socks, and leave overnight. The pressure and heat will help the cream or oil penetrate deep into the skin.

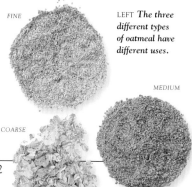

FINE

LEFT *The three different types of oatmeal have different uses.*

MEDIUM

LEFT *Wear socks for a few hours after exfoliating with oatmeal.*

COARSE

Witch hazel

HAMAMELIS VIRGINIANA

BENEFITS
Anti-
inflammatory
Antiseptic
Astringent
Toning

A SHRUBBY PLANT *of the Hamamelis species, witch hazel has been distilled and used for centuries for its rejuvenating properties. It is good for oily skin, as well as in soothing body preparations.*

BEAUTY RECIPES

☙ For oily skin, dilute 1 part distilled witch hazel to 2 parts water to make a toner. Use after cleansing and before moisturizing.

☙ For an oily scalp, mix 1 part distilled witch hazel with 4 parts water and dab on the scalp with a cotton ball. If your scalp is very oily, repeat each time you shampoo.

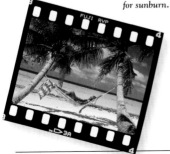

BELOW **Witch hazel is particularly soothing for sunburn.**

☙ For a soothing, rejuvenating, antiwrinkle mask, combine 1 tsp (5 ml) each of distilled witch hazel, cider vinegar, and apricot-kernel oil, with 1 egg yolk and 1 tsp (5 ml) of lemon juice. Blend all the ingredients together, apply to the face and neck, and leave on for 10 to 15 minutes before rinsing with warm water. This mixture will keep for several days in the refrigerator.

☙ To ease sunburn, moisten a cloth or cotton ball with witch hazel and gently apply to affected areas.

☙ To treat cold sores, dab on witch hazel daily to promote healing.

ABOVE **Leaves of the witch hazel, a common shrub like tree.**

APRICOT-KERNEL OIL

Aloe vera

ALOE BARBADENSIS

ALOE LEAVES

BENEFITS

Astringent

Rejuvenating

Softening

Soothing

THE ALOE VERA PLANT *produces a gel and a juice that are widely used in beauty preparations. Aloe vera helps to draw out infection and heals skin irritations. It helps combat wrinkles and can heal sunburn.*

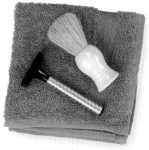

ABOVE **Aloe vera can help heal shaving cuts or abrasions.**

Aloe vera can be easily grown as a houseplant. Its fleshy leaves contain the gel. Break open the leaf and use directly on the skin.

❋ To ease cracked and sore lips, apply aloe juice daily.

❋ To soothe dry, sensitive, or irritated skin, apply fresh gel directly onto the skin.

❋ To help heal any cuts or scratches caused by the razor, apply a little aloe vera gel after shaving.

BEAUTY RECIPES

❋ To treat acne, apply enough aloe vera juice to cover the affected area. Leave for 10 minutes before rinsing. Apply daily. Skin may become dry, but only initially.

❋ For a marvelous skin tonic, smooth a little fresh juice over the face and leave for 15 minutes before rinsing.

RIGHT
Aloe vera is a well-known succulent plant.

> CAUTION
>
> Do not use aloe vera during pregnancy or when breast-feeding.

Common beauty problems

MANY BEAUTY PROBLEMS *can be easily dealt with at home, and the most common are listed below. If you are particularly concerned about a persistent complaint, consult a qualified therapist or your physician.*

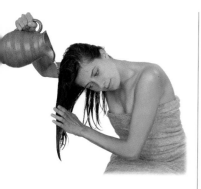

DRY HAIR

Massage olive or wheat-germ oil into the scalp (*see pages 17 and 47*). Mashed banana and grapeseed oil can be used in the same way (*see page 27*). See also Eggs (*page 50*) and Almond (*page 35*).

DULL OR DAMAGED HAIR

Apply mashed avocado and lemon juice (*see page 28*). Use an infusion of rosemary as a tonic and to condition dark hair (*see page 44*). Use diluted apple cider vinegar to enhance fair hair (*see page 49*).

DANDRUFF

Massage lemon or apple juice (*see pages 37 and 31*), an infusion of rosemary (*see page 44*), or olive oil (*see page 17*) into the scalp. Use apple cider vinegar as a final rinse after washing (*see page 49*). See also Tea tree (*page 41*).

OILY HAIR

Use lemon juice diluted with distilled water as a rinse (*see page 37*).

FLYAWAY HAIR

Apply a conditioner made from combining natural yogurt and a whole egg (*see page 51*).

BRITTLE HAIR

Apply a paste of mashed banana and grapeseed oil and wrap in a warm towel (*see page 27*).

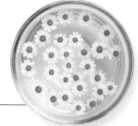

PUFFY, SWOLLEN, OR TIRED EYES

Place cold chamomile or rosemary tea bags on each closed eye to relax and revive them (*see pages 45 and 44*). Slices of cucumber, papaya, and potato are also useful. Alternatively, cup the hands over closed eyes and rest for 20 minutes. *See also Fennel (page 43).*

WRINKLES

Smooth fresh aloe vera juice over the face daily (*see page 54*). Use a mask made with witch hazel, cider vinegar, egg yolk, lemon, and apricot-kernel oil (*see page 53*). *See also Apricot (page 36) and Fennel (page 43).*

PIMPLES

Treat with grated carrot and lemon juice (*see page 34*), witch hazel (*see page 53*), or lavender water (*see page 46*). Dab neat tea tree or lavender oil onto pimples (*see pages 41 and 46*). *See also Potato (page 33).*

ACNE

Apply apple pulp (*see page 31*). Use cucumber and lemon juice as an astringent (*see page 32*). Add lavender, juniper, or sandalwood essential oils to a facial sauna. Dab with aloe vera juice or tea tree essential oil (*see pages 54 and 41*). *See also Papaya (page 29) Peppermint (page 40), and Pineapple (page 30).*

BLACKHEADS

Add chamomile flowers to boiling water for a facial sauna (*see page 45*). See also *Tea tree (page 41).*

COLD SORES

Apply neat witch hazel or tea tree essential oil daily (*see pages 53 and 41*).

CRACKED SORE LIPS

Use honey combined with a little rose water as a lip balm (*see page 48*), or apply aloe vera juice daily (*see page 54*).

WEAK NAILS

Massage wheat-germ oil into the cuticles (*see page 47*).

CHAPPED SKIN

Massage with lavender and almond oil (*see page 46*), or add a few drops of sandalwood essential oil to bathwater (*see page 38*).

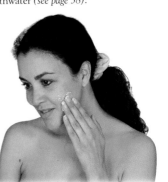

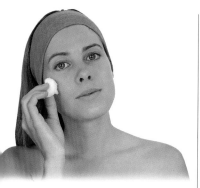

OILY SKIN

Apply pineapple skins (*see page 30*). Use lemon juice or witch hazel diluted with water as a toner (*see pages 37 and 53*). Massage with geranium, sandalwood, or lavender essential oils blended with a carrier oil (*see pages 39, 38, and 46*). Use juniper essential oil in a facial sauna (*see page 42*). Apply a mask made with egg, yogurt, and oatmeal (*see page 51*). See also Rosemary (*page 44*).

DRY SKIN

Mashed banana and avocado are the basis of useful preparations (*see pages 27 and 28*). Carrot oil diluted in a carrier oil makes an effective moisturizer (*see page 34*). Use a mask made with egg yolk, wheat-germ oil, and honey (*see page 50*). Add oatmeal to bathwater (*see page 52*). Use a few drops of chamomile essential oil in the bathwater (*see page 45*). See also Almond (*page 35*), Aloe vera (*page 54*), Apricot (*page 36*).

DULL OR PALE SKIN

Use a massage paste made with ground almonds and almond oil (*see page 35*).

IRRITATED SKIN

Chamomile essential oil is useful for skin that is sensitive, dry, or itchy (*see page 45*). Use in the bath, in a massage blend or add to natural creams.

SENSITIVE SKIN

Use rose water (*page 25*) and wheat-germ oil (*page 47*).

FLAKY SKIN

Apply a scrub made with ground almonds (*see page 35*). Alternatively you can also apply a face mask made from mashed papaya and honey (*see page 29*).

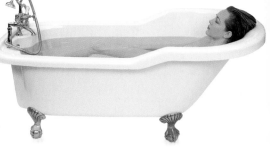

BLEMISHED AND SCARRED SKIN
Massage wheat-germ oil into the skin nightly (see page 47).

DISCOLORED SKIN
Smooth yogurt and cider vinegar (see page 51), or lemon juice (see page 37), into the skin.

HARD SKIN
Use a mixture of yogurt and cider vinegar (see page 51), or use lemon halves (see page 37). For hands and feet specifically, see also Pineapple (page 30) and Lavender (page 46).

ROUGH SKIN
Rub the insides of avocado skins over the affected area (see page 28). For the hands specifically, massage in almond oil mixed with a few drops of lavender essential oil (see page 46).

ITCHY SKIN
Use chamomile essential oil in bathwater (see page 45).

SUNBURN
Apply grated carrot (see page 34), or plain, live yogurt mixed with rose water (see page 51). Apple, cucumber, or potato slices can be applied to burnt areas (see pages 31, 32 and 33).

WARTS
Bind a fresh piece of pineapple to the wart with gauze (see page 30).

INFLAMED COMPLEXION
Blend the juice of raw potatoes with oatmeal to make a face pack (see page 33).

ACHING MUSCLES
Massage a combination of peppermint and grapeseed oil or lavender essential oil into the affected area (see pages 40 and 46).

CELLULITE
Make up a massage oil with lemon, fennel, rosemary, geranium, or juniper essential oils in a carrier oil (see page 16). Add drops of the same essential oils to the bathwater. Drink fennel tea (see page 43).

WATER RETENTION
Add juniper essential oil to a bath before a menstrual period (see page 42).

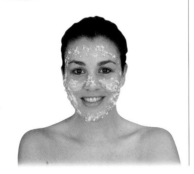

Further reading

THE COMPLETE ILLUSTRATED GUIDE
TO AROMATHERAPY by *Julia Lawless*
(Element Books, 1997)

THE COMPLETE ILLUSTRATED GUIDE
TO MASSAGE by *Stewart Mitchell*
(Element Books, 1997)

THE COMPLETE ILLUSTRATED GUIDE
TO NUTRITIONAL HEALING by *Denise
Mortimore* (Element Books, 1998)

HEALTH ESSENTIALS: NATURAL
BEAUTY by *Sidra Shaukat* (Element
Books, 1996)

MAKING YOUR OWN COSMETICS by
Neal's Yard Remedies (Aurum Press,
1997)

IN A NUTSHELL: HERBAL MEDICINE
by *Non Shaw* (Element Books, 1998)

Useful addresses

**National Herbalists
Association of Australia**
Montville Road
Mapleton
Queensland
Australia 4560

The Herb Society of South Africa
P.O. Box 5783
Durban
Republic of South Africa 4000

Neal's Yard Remedies
15 Neal's Yard
Covent Garden
London WC2H 9DP
U K

**Joy of Life (Aromatherapy
and Natural Beauty)**
280 Balham High Road
London SW17 7AL
U K

Ledet Oils
P.O. Box 2354
Fair Oaks
CA 95628
USA

Aroma Vera Inc.
1830 S. Robertson Blvd. #203,
Los Angeles
CA 90035
USA

*Other step-by-step guides
in the Nutshell Series*

ALEXANDER TECHNIQUE

ALTERNATIVE MEDICINE

AROMATHERAPY

BACH FLOWER REMEDIES

BIORHYTHMS

CHINESE HERBAL MEDICINE

HERBAL MEDICINE

HOMEOPATHY

MASSAGE

NATURAL HOME REMEDIES

REFLEXOLOGY

SHIATSU

VITAMINS AND MINERALS

YOGA